Busy Body, Balanced Life

Ultimate Nutrition and Fitness Hacks for Professionals On The Move

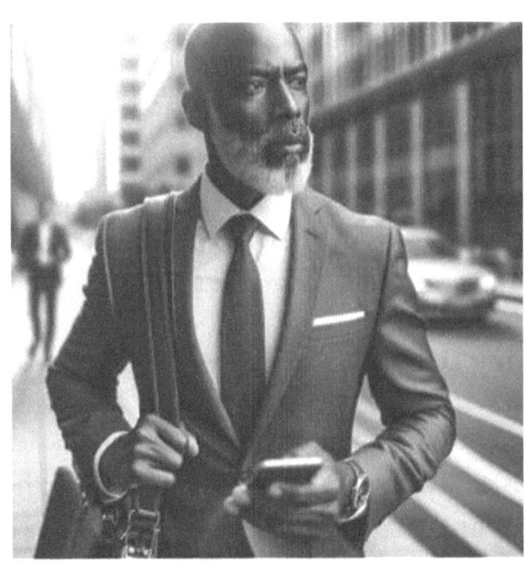

'Denike Owolabi

Busy Body, Balanced Life

Ordering Details

To place orders or for details of discounts for bulk purchases by organizations or groups either for support, gift, training packages, fundraising, or any other educational purposes, send an email to denikeowolabi65@gmail.com.

Table of Contents

Introduction

Welcome to Busy Body, Balanced Life: Nutrition and Fitness Hacks for Professionals on the Move! I am thrilled to have you here, joining me on this journey towards a healthier and more balanced lifestyle. As a passionate fitness enthusiast and advocate for well-being, I understand the demands and challenges that come with a hectic professional life.

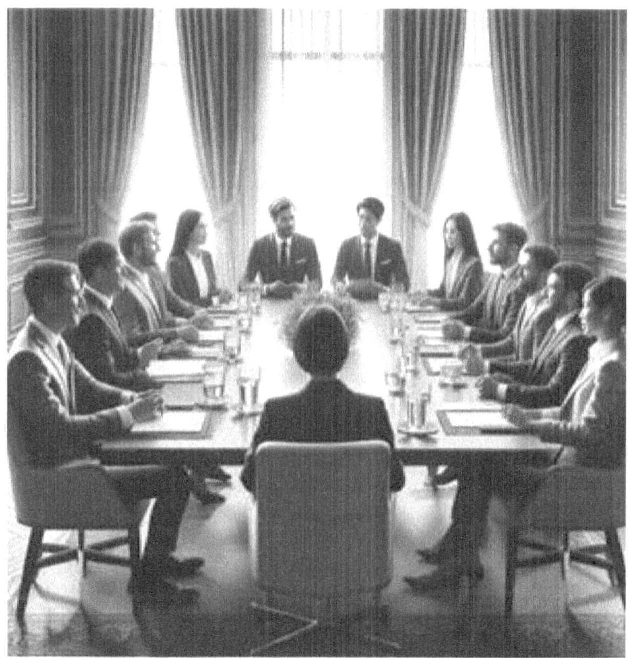

In the fast-paced world we live in, it's easy to let our

health take a backseat as we juggle countless responsibilities. The constant struggle to find time for exercise and maintain a nutritious diet can be overwhelming. However, it is precisely during these busy moments that prioritising our physical and mental well-being becomes even more crucial.

This e-book is designed to empower busy professionals like you with practical strategies, time-saving tips, and invaluable insights to achieve a healthier and more fulfilling life. We will

delve into the correlation between nutrition, fitness, and productivity, recognising that nourishing our bodies and staying active play pivotal roles in enhancing our performance both at work and in our personal lives.

Throughout the chapters, we will explore the common obstacles faced by busy professionals in their pursuit of fitness and proper nutrition. From the temptations of sedentary habits to the allure of quick, unhealthy snacks, we will address these challenges head-on and arm you with actionable solutions.

In Chapter 2, we will learn about fueling our bodies for success, discovering quick and wholesome breakfast options, smart snacking strategies to avoid energy crashes, and effective ways to plan and prepare nutritious lunches that keep us energized throughout the day.

Chapter 3 will highlight the importance of staying hydrated and making healthy beverage choices, unveiling how proper hydration can positively impact your performance and overall well-being.

In Chapter 4, we will dive into the realm of mindful eating and explore its potential to reduce stress and prevent overeating. As busy professionals, understanding the connection between our emotional state and eating habits can empower us to make more mindful choices.

Making fitness a part of your daily routine can be challenging, but fret not! In Chapter 5, we will explore creative strategies to integrate physical activity into your workday and to turn household chores into exercise opportunities.

Finally, in the concluding chapter, we will share final thoughts and motivations and emphasize the significance of taking small steps towards a healthier lifestyle. Remember, progress is about consistency, not perfection, and every positive change you make contributes to your overall well-being

I am excited for you to embark on this

transformative journey with me, armed with newfound knowledge and empowered to make positive changes in your life. So, let's dive in and start prioritising our health and happiness amidst the demands of a busy professional life.

Let's unlock your potential and discover the best version of yourself - a healthier, fitter, and more vibrant you!

Let's get started!

Chapter 1:

Understanding the Lifestyle of the Professional on the Move

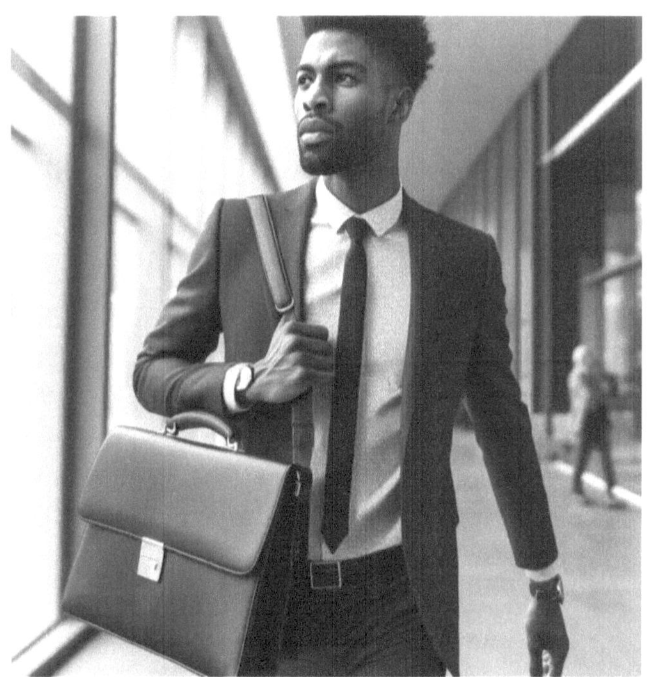

In our fast-paced modern world, being a busy professional is more than just a job – it's a lifestyle that demands unwavering dedication and constant multitasking. As we strive for success and navigate the challenges of our careers, we often find ourselves entangled in a web of responsibilities, deadlines, and commitments that leave little time for anything else.

Unfortunately, amidst the hustle and bustle, our health and well-being often take a backseat, leading to adverse consequences that we may not immediately recognise.

Embracing the busy lifestyle

The busy professional lifestyle is characterised by ambition, long working hours, and a drive to achieve our goals. Embracing this lifestyle is a testament to our determination and passion for what we do. However, it's essential to strike a balance between pursuing our ambitions and taking care of ourselves. Recognising the value of a healthy and fit body will not only enhance our performance in the workplace but also contribute to a more fulfilling and sustainable journey.

The Tug-of-war: work and personal life

One of the most significant challenges faced by busy professionals is the constant tug-of-war between work and personal life. Striking the right balance becomes a delicate art, as we try to excel in our careers without compromising the time we spend with loved ones or nurturing our passions outside of work. Understanding this delicate interplay is vital for maintaining overall well-being and avoiding the pitfalls of burnout.

Prioritisation and time management

In the midst of endless to-do lists and hectic schedules, effective prioritisation and time management become invaluable skills. As busy professionals, we need to identify what truly matters to us and allocate time accordingly. Making health and well-being a top priority is not just a luxury but a necessity, as it lays the foundation for sustained success in both our professional and personal lives.

The hidden toll of stress

Stress is an ever-present companion in the lives of busy professionals. While a certain level of stress can be motivating and propel us forward, chronic stress can take a toll on our mental and physical health. Understanding the impact of stress on our well-being is essential to implement coping mechanisms and stress-reduction strategies that help us thrive in the face of challenges.

The sedentary trap

The nature of many professions often involves

prolonged hours of sitting, whether at a desk, during meetings, or during long commutes. This sedentary lifestyle can have adverse effects on our health, contributing to issues such as back pain, weight gain, and reduced cardiovascular fitness. Learning to break free from the sedentary trap is vital for improving our overall health and vitality.

Cultivating a mind-set for health and wellness

To make sustainable changes, we must cultivate a mind-set that prioritises health and wellness. This involves recognising that our well-being is an essential aspect of our success, happiness, and overall quality of life. By viewing health as an investment rather than an expense, we can approach fitness and nutrition with the dedication and enthusiasm that fuels our professional endeavours.

Conclusion:

Understanding the busy professional lifestyle is the first step toward achieving a harmonious balance between our career aspirations and our health and well-being. By recognising the challenges, embracing prioritisation, and cultivating a proactive mind-set, we can navigate this demanding lifestyle with grace and resilience.

In the subsequent chapters of this e-book, we will explore practical strategies for integrating fitness and nutrition seamlessly into our busy lives, empowering us to thrive both professionally and personally. Remember, your health is your most valuable asset – let's embark on this journey together towards a healthier, more fulfilled you.

Chapter 2

Fuelling Your Body for Success

In the fast-paced world of busy professionals, success often hinges on our ability to perform at our best day in and day out. The key to sustained success lies not only in our skills and dedication but also in how we fuel our bodies to meet the demands of our dynamic lives.

Nutrition plays a pivotal role in providing the energy, focus, and resilience needed to excel in our careers and personal pursuits. In this chapter, we will delve into the critical role of nutrition and explore practical strategies to fuel our body for success.

The role of nutrition in energy and productivity

The food we consume is the fuel that powers our bodies and minds. Understanding the intricate relationship between nutrition, energy levels, and productivity is essential for optimizing performance.

Nutrition plays a critical role in maintaining energy levels and enhancing productivity in individuals. The food we consume provides the necessary nutrients that fuel our bodies and support various physiological processes essential for optimal performance. Whether it is in the workplace, at school, or during everyday tasks, a well-balanced diet can significantly impact our ability to stay focused, alert, and productive.

A well-balanced diet rich in carbohydrates, proteins, and fats supports energy metabolism, ensuring a steady supply of fuel for both physical and mental tasks. Essential nutrients like omega-3 fatty acids and B-vitamins aid brain function, focus, and concentration, while stable blood sugar levels prevent fatigue and cognitive impairment. Additionally, good nutrition strengthens the immune system, promotes physical endurance, and enhances overall mood and well-being.

By prioritising nutrition, busy professionals can unlock their full potential and maintain peak productivity in their demanding lives.

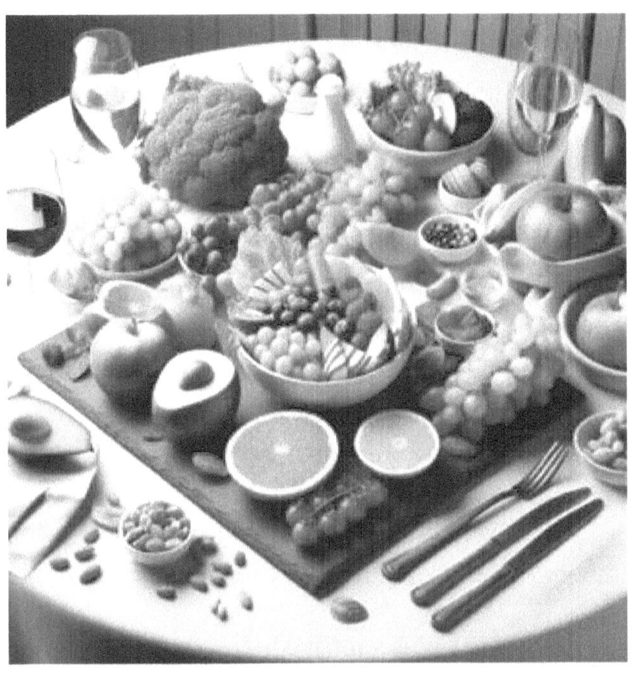

In summary, nutrition plays a vital role in sustaining energy levels, mental clarity, and overall productivity. A balanced diet that includes a variety of nutrient-dense foods supports energy metabolism, brain function, focus, immune system, and physical endurance. Moreover, recognising the connection between nutrition and productivity underscores the importance of investing in proper nutrition education and initiatives to promote well-being in various aspects of life.

Rise and shine: Quick and healthy breakfast options

Breakfast is often hailed as the most important meal of the day, setting the tone for our energy levels and focus.

It provides the necessary energy to kick-start our mornings and fuel our bodies for the day ahead. However, in our fast-paced lives, finding time to prepare a nutritious breakfast can be a challenge.

In a nutshell, for busy professionals, starting the day with a balanced and nutritious breakfast is vital.

Here are some quick and healthy breakfast options that will keep you energized and ready to tackle whatever comes your way.

1. Overnight Oats: Prepare a delicious and nutritious breakfast the night before by combining rolled oats with your choice of milk (dairy or plant-based) in a jar. Add toppings like fresh fruits, nuts, and a drizzle of honey or maple syrup. Refrigerate overnight, and in the morning, your oats will be ready to eat, no cooking required.

2. Smoothie bowl: Blend together your favourite fruits, leafy greens (such as spinach

or kale), Greek yogurt, and a splash of liquid (water, milk, or juice) to create a thick and creamy smoothie. Pour it into a bowl and top with granola, chia seeds, and additional fruits for addedtexture and nutrients.

3. Avocado toast: Mash ripe avocado onto whole-grain toast and sprinkle with a pinch of salt and pepper. For added protein, top with sliced hard-boiled eggs, smoked salmon, or crumbled feta cheese. Avocado toast is not only quick to make but also a great source of healthy fats and fibre.

4. Greek yogurt parfait: Layer Greek yogurt with fresh berries, nuts, and a drizzle of honey in a glass or jar to create a visually appealing and nutritious parfait. Greek yogurt is rich in protein, while berries provide antioxidants and fibre.

5. Chia seed pudding: Mix chia seeds with your choice of milk and sweetener (such as honey or agave syrup) in a jar. Let it sit in the refrigerator overnight, and in the morning, you will have a creamy and nutrient-packed pudding. Top with fruits and nuts for added flavour and texture.

6. Veggie omelette: Whisk together eggs or egg whites and pour them into a heated, non-stick pan. Add chopped vegetables like bell peppers, tomatoes, spinach, and mushrooms. Cook until the omelette sets, then fold it in half. This protein-packed breakfast will keep you satisfied until lunch.

7. Whole grain cereals: Choose a whole-grain cereal with low added sugar and pair it with your choice of milk or yogurt. Top with sliced bananas, berries, or a sprinkle of nuts for added nutrients and crunch.

Remember, a healthy breakfast doesn't have to be time-consuming. With a little planning and creativity, you can enjoy a quick and nutritious meal to fuel your day and set a positive tone for healthy eating habits throughout the day.

Smart snacking strategies to avoid rnergy crashes

In the midst of a busy workday, it's easy to succumb to the allure of sugary or processed snacks for a quick energy boost. However, these choices often lead to energy crashes and decreased productivity.

So, snacking can either be a helpful tool to maintain energy levels throughout the day or a pitfall leading to energy crashes and poor productivity.

Making smart snacking choices is crucial to keep your energy steady and your focus sharp. We will explore smart snacking alternatives that stabilize blood sugar levels and provide lasting nourishment to keep you energized throughout the day.

Smart snacking strategies to avoid energy crashes

1. Opt for nutrient-dense snacks: Choose snacks that provide essential nutrients to fuel your body and brain. Include a combination of macronutrients (carbohydrates, proteins, and fats) and micronutrients (vitamins and minerals) in your snacks. Examples of nutrient-dense snacks include whole fruits, nuts, Greek yogurt, and whole-grain crackers with cheese.

2. Choose complex carbohydrates: Snacks rich in complex carbohydrates, such as whole grains, fruits, and vegetables, provide a steady release of glucose, helping to sustain energy levels without causing rapid spikes and crashes in blood sugar. Avoid snacks with refined sugars and processed carbohydrates, which can lead to quick

energy highs followed by crashes.

3. Include protein: Protein is essential for maintaining energy and promoting feelings of fullness. Protein-rich snacks can help stabilize blood sugar levels and provide a sustained source of energy. Consider options like boiled eggs, lean turkey slices, or nut butter with whole-grain toast.

4. Mind the portion sizes: Be mindful of portion sizes when snacking. Overeating, even with healthy snacks, can lead to feelings of sluggishness and reduced energy levels. Use small containers or bags to pack controlled portions and prevent mindless munching.

5. Stay hydrated: Dehydration can contribute to feelings of fatigue. Keep a water bottle nearby and drink water regularly throughout the day. If you prefer flavoured beverages, opt for herbal teas or infuse your water with slices of fruits for a refreshing twist.

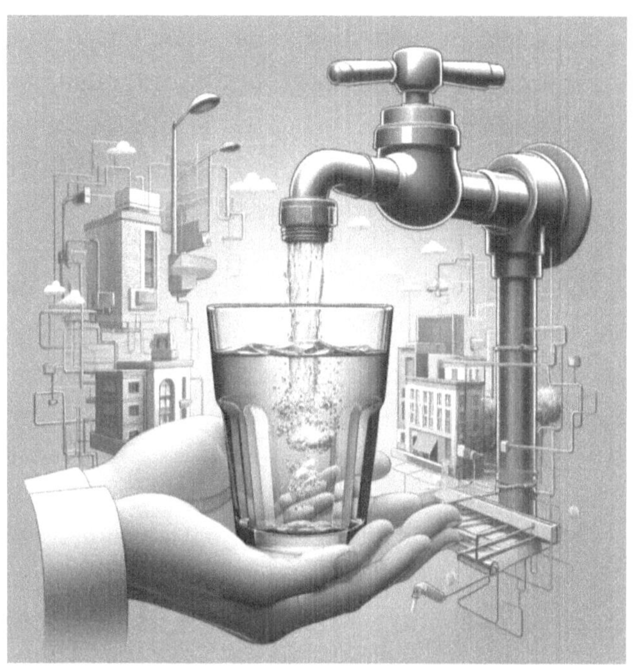

6. Plan ahead: Prepare your snacks in advance, especially if you have a busy schedule. Having healthy snacks readily available will prevent you from reaching for unhealthy options when hunger strikes.

7. Avoid processed and sugary snacks: Processed snacks high in unhealthy fats, added sugars, and empty calories can lead to energy crashes. Instead, focus on whole, natural foods that provide sustained energy and nourishment.

8. Listen to your body: Pay attention to your body's hunger cues and avoid mindless snacking. Sometimes, the feeling of fatigue may be a signal that you need a short break or a quick stretch rather than a snack.

9. Time your snacks: Snack strategically between meals to maintain consistent energy levels. Aim for snacks about halfway between breakfast and lunch, and again between lunch and dinner.

10. Combine snacks with physical activity: Instead of reaching for a snack when you feel a dip in energy, consider taking a short walk or doing some light stretching. Physical activity can naturally boost your energy and improve productivity.

In summary, by adopting these smart snacking strategies, you can avoid energy crashes and stay alert and productive throughout the day. Remember, snacking should complement your main meals and provide nourishment to help you perform at your best.

Navigating nutritious lunches at work

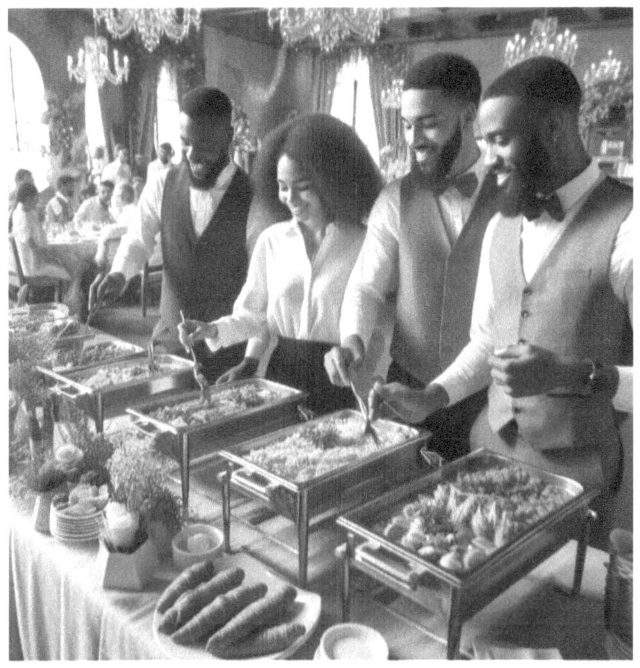

Maintaining a healthy and nutritious diet during work hours is essential for sustaining energy levels, enhancing productivity, and promoting overall well-being. However, navigating lunch choices at work can be challenging, with temptations like fast-food options and office snacks readily available.

Here are some strategies to help you make healthier lunch choices and ensure your midday meal supports your health and productivity:

1. Pack your lunch: Preparing your lunch at home gives you control over the ingredients and portion sizes. Aim for a balanced meal that includes lean proteins (such as grilled chicken, tofu, or beans), whole grains(brown rice, quinoa, or whole-grain bread), and a variety of colourful vegetables. Packing your lunch also saves time and money, making it a win-win choice.

2. Seek out healthy options: If you prefer to buy lunch at work, look for restaurants or cafes that offer nutritious choices. Opt for salads with a variety of vegetables, lean proteins, and healthy fats like avocado or nuts. Choose whole-grain wraps or sandwiches instead of those made with refined white bread.

3. Mindful portion control: Even when choosing healthy options, be mindful of portion sizes. Overeating, even with nutritious foods, can lead to feelings of lethargy and decreased productivity. Listen to your body's hunger cues and stop eating when you feel comfortably satisfied.

4. Plan ahead for work events: Office gatherings or business lunches can often

involve tempting but unhealthy foods. Plan ahead by eating a nutritious snack before the event, so you're not overly hungry and tempted to indulge in unhealthy choices. Look for healthier options on the menu, and focus on moderation if treats are available.

5. Be wary of hidden calories: Be cautious of condiments, dressings, and sauces that can add hidden calories and unhealthy fats to your meals.

6. Practice mindful eating: Take the time to enjoy your lunch away from your desk. Mindful eating allows you to savour your food, be aware of your hunger and fullness cues, and promotes better digestion.

In summary, by adopting these strategies and making conscious choices about your lunch at work, you can support your health and well-being, boost productivity, and feel energized throughout the day.

The impact of evening nutrition on restful sleep

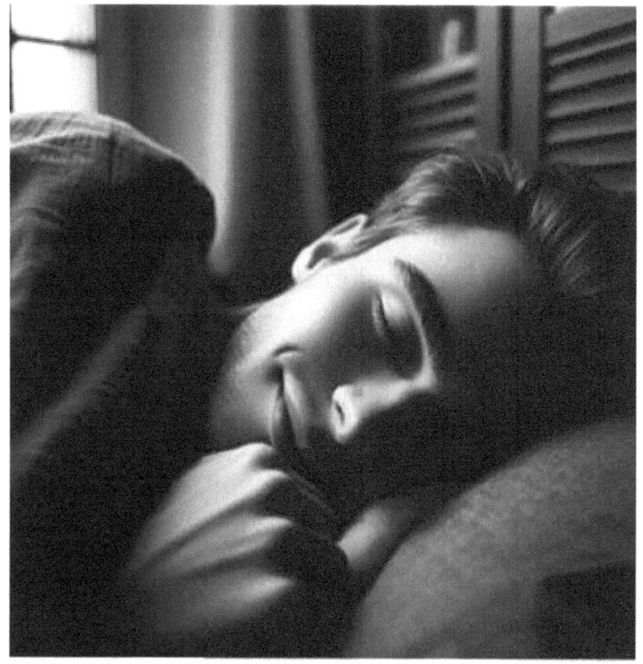

The busy professionals' lifestyle often extends into the evening hours, impacting on sleep quality. The relationship between nutrition and sleep is a complex and essential aspect of overall health and well-being.

It is important you are aware that specific food choices can positively or negatively influence the quality of your rest and a quality rest is vital for recharging and rejuvenating your body and mind.

1. Digestion and sleep: Eating a large, heavy meal close to bedtime can disrupt the body's natural sleep-wake cycle. When we eat, our bodies direct blood flow to the digestive system to process the food. This can interfere with the relaxation response needed for falling asleep and achieving deep, restorative sleep.

2. Avoid heavy, fatty foods: High-fat and greasy foods, such as fried dishes and fatty meats, are more challenging to digest and can lead to discomfort and indigestion, making it difficult to fall asleep and stay asleep.

3. Caffeine and stimulants: Consuming caffeine and other stimulants in the evening can disrupt sleep patterns, leading to difficulties falling asleep or staying asleep. Be mindful of hidden sources of caffeine, such as chocolate and some medications.

4. Limit fluid intake: Drinking too much liquid close to bedtime may lead to frequent trips to the bathroom during the night, disrupting sleep continuity. While staying hydrated is essential, try to consume most of your fluids earlier in the evening.

5. Promote serotonin production: Serotonin is a neurotransmitter that promotes relaxation and sleepiness. Foods rich in tryptophan, an amino acid that helps produce serotonin, can be beneficial in the evening. These include nuts, seeds, and bananas.

6. Melatonin Boosters: Melatonin is a hormone that regulates sleep-wake cycles. Some foods, like tart cherries, kiwis, and tomatoes, naturally contain melatonin or compounds that help boost its production, potentially aiding in sleep quality.

7. Balance carbohydrates: Eating balanced meals with moderate carbohydrates can help promote sleep. Carbohydrates trigger the release of insulin, which facilitates the entry of tryptophan into the brain, promoting relaxation and sleepiness.

8. Control sugar intake: While carbohydrates are beneficial for sleep, consuming sugary foods and beverages in the evening can cause blood sugar spikes and crashes, leading to sleep disturbances.

9. Avoid excessive alcohol: Although alcohol may initially induce drowsiness, it disrupts

the sleep cycle and can lead to fragmented and less restful sleep. If you choose not to avoid alcohol (not recommended), it's best to limit it's intake in the evening.

10. Time your meals: Aim to eat your evening meal at least a few hours before bedtime. This allows ample time for digestion before lying down to sleep.

11. Listen to your body: Pay attention to how certain foods affect your sleep. Everyone's metabolism is different, so it's essential to notice any patterns between your evening nutrition and the quality of your sleep.

12. Create a relaxing bedtime routine: In addition to eating the right foods, establish a soothing bedtime routine to signal to your body that it's time to wind down and prepare for sleep. This can include activities like reading, gentle stretching, or meditation.

In conclusion, what we eat in the evening can significantly impact our sleep quality.

Fuelling your body for success is not just about grabbing a quick bite to eat; it's about making intentional and nutritious choices that support your performance and well-being.

By making conscious choices about the foods you consume before bedtime, you will not only create a supportive environment for restorative sleep and wake up feeling refreshed and energized each morning but also set yourself up for sustained success in your professional and personal endeavours.

Chapter 3

Staying Hydrated and Healthy

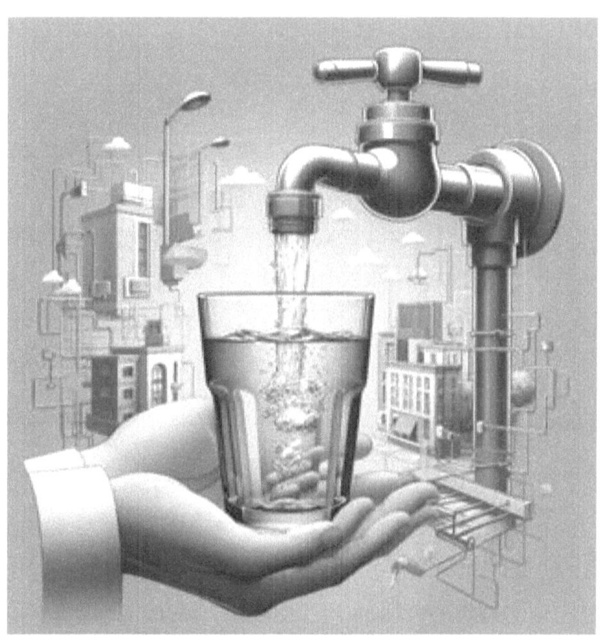

The importance of proper hydration for optimal performance

Water, the elixir of life, is the foundation of vitality and plays a central role in maintaining our overall health and well-being. Staying hydrated is a fundamental aspect of optimal performance and well-being.

Proper hydration is essential for numerous bodily functions, and its impact on our physical and mental vitality cannot be overstated.

Here are why staying hydrated is crucial for optimal health and vitality:

1. Essential for body functions: Water is a fundamental component of every cell, tissue, and organ in our bodies. It aids in various physiological processes, including digestion, nutrient absorption, circulation, and temperature regulation. When we are well-hydrated, our bodies can function efficiently, ensuring we feel energized and vibrant.

2. Sustains energy levels: Dehydration can lead to feelings of fatigue and decreased energy levels. When we don't consume enough water, our blood volume decreases, causing the heart to work harder to pump oxygen and nutrients to our organs and muscles. Proper hydration helps maintain adequate blood flow, supporting energy and endurance throughout the day.

3. Mental clarity and focus: Staying hydrated is crucial for maintaining cognitive function.

Research shows that even mild dehydration can impair memory, attention, and decision-making abilities. By drinking enough water, we can keep our minds sharp, improve concentration, and enhance overall mental performance.

4. Aids digestion and detoxification: Water is vital for proper digestion and the absorption of nutrients. It helps break down food and move it through the digestive tract smoothly. Additionally, staying hydrated supports kidney function, allowing the body to effectively eliminate waste and toxins through urine.

5. Supports physical performance: Whether you're an athlete or engage in regular physical activity, staying hydrated is vital for performance and recovery. Dehydration can lead to reduced endurance, muscle cramps, and increased risk of heat-related injuries. Proper hydration helps optimize physical performance and aids in post-exercise recovery.

6. Regulates body temperature: Water acts as a natural coolant, helping to regulate body temperature through sweat. During hot

weather or intense physical activity, our bodies release sweat to cool down. Replenishing lost fluids through proper hydration is essential to prevent heat-related illnesses.

7. Promotes healthy skin: Adequate hydration is essential for maintaining healthy and glowing skin. Water helps moisturize the skin from the inside out, reducing dryness and promoting a radiant complexion.

8. Weight management: Staying hydrated can support weight management efforts. Sometimes, thirst can be mistaken for hunger, leading to unnecessary snacking and calorie intake. Drinking water before meals can help control appetite and promote a feeling of fullness, leading to reduced calorie consumption.

9. Boosts immune function: Water plays an important role in supporting a healthy immune system. It assists in the production and transport of immune cells throughout the body, helping to defend against infections and illnesses.

To stay adequately hydrated, it is generally

recommended to drink about eight glasses of water per day, though individual needs may vary based on factors such as climate, activity level, and overall health. Remember that other beverages and water-rich foods, such as fruits and vegetables, also contribute to your daily hydration needs.

Practical tips for staying hydrated throughout the day:

1. Carry a water bottle: Keep a reusable water bottle with you at all times. Having water readily available makes it easier to sip throughout the day, reminding you to stay hydrated. Get into the habit of refilling your bottle during lunchtime.

2. Set reminders: Use your phone or computer to set hourly reminders to drink water. These gentle nudges will help you establish a hydration routine.

3. Flavour your water: If you find plain water boring, add natural flavours like lemon, cucumber, mint, or berries to enhance the taste and make drinking water more enjoyable.

4. Track your intake: Use a water tracking app or a simple journal to record your water

consumption. Seeing your progress can be motivating and help you reach your daily hydration goals.

5. Start and end with water: Begin your day by drinking a glass of warm water as soon as you wake up. Also, make it a habit to drink a glass of water before each meal to help control appetite and ensure you get enough fluids.

6. Hydrate with herbal teas: Herbal teas are a great alternative to water and can add variety to your hydration routine. Opt for caffeine-free options like chamomile, peppermint, or hibiscus.

7. Snack on water-rich foods: Incorporate fruits and vegetables with high water content into your diet, such as watermelon, cucumber, oranges, and celery. These foods contribute to your hydration needs.

8. Use a straw: Drinking through a straw can help you consume more water without even realizing it. It's a simple trick to encourage more sipping throughout the day.

9. Hydrate before and after exercise: Drink water before, during, and after physical

activity to replenish lost fluids and prevent dehydration.

10. Stay hydrated in hot weather: Increase your water intake during hot weather or if you engage in outdoor activities to prevent heat-related dehydration.

11. Limit dehydrating beverages: Minimise the consumption of dehydrating drinks like alcohol and caffeinated beverages. If you do consume them, balance them with extra water intake.

12. Hydration as a family: Encourage your family members or co-workers to stay hydrated together. Creating a supportive environment can make it easier to maintain good habits.

Remember that individual hydration needs may vary based on factors like age, activity level, and climate. Pay attention to your body's signals and adjust your water intake accordingly.

By incorporating these practical tips into your daily routine, you can stay hydrated, feel refreshed, and maintain optimal health and vitality.

In conclusion, water is the cornerstone of vitality,

impacting nearly every aspect of our physical and mental well-being. By prioritising hydration and making conscious efforts to drink enough water each day, we can unlock our full potential, feel revitalised, and enjoy a vibrant and energised life.

Healthy beverage options for busy professionals

1. Water: The simplest and most essential beverage for staying hydrated throughout the day remains water.

2. Herbal teas: Herbal teas, such as chamomile, peppermint, and rooibos, are caffeine-free and can be both soothing and hydrating. Enjoy a warm cup during breaks to relax and refresh.

3. Green tea: For a mild caffeine boost without the jitters, green tea is an excellent option. It contains antioxidants and has been linked to various health benefits.

4. Sparkling water: If you crave carbonation, opt for plain sparkling water or add a splash of fresh fruit juice for a naturally flavoured and refreshing drink.

5. Coconut water: Coconut water is a natural

electrolyte-rich beverage that can help replenish nutrients after physical activity or during busy days.

6. Vegetable juices: Freshly squeezed vegetable juices, like carrot or celery juice, are nutrient-dense options that provide vitamins and minerals while avoiding added sugars.

7. Smoothies: Blend together fruits, vegetables, and protein sources like Greek yogurt or plant-based protein powder to create a nutritious and portable smoothie. Prepare it in advance and take it with you to work.

8. Iced herbal infusions: Brew herbal teas and let them cool in the refrigerator for a refreshing and hydrating iced beverage without added sugars or artificial flavors.

9. Homemade infused water: Infuse water with slices of fruits like lemon, cucumber, strawberries, or mint leaves for a naturally flavoured beverage without added sugars or artificial sweeteners.

10. Almond milk or oat milk: For a dairy-free alternative to milk, try almond milk or oat milk. Look for unsweetened varieties to

avoid added sugars.

Remember that portion control is key, even with healthy beverages. Avoid excessive consumption of sugary or caffeinated drinks, and opt for more hydrating options throughout the day. By making conscious choices about your beverage intake, you can stay refreshed, energized, and focused, supporting your productivity as a busy professional.

Chapter 4

Mindful Eating for Stress Reduction

The connection between stress and eating habits:

Stress can significantly impact eating habits, leading to emotional eating, cravings for unhealthy foods, and changes in appetite.

Many individuals turn to comfort foods as a coping mechanism during stressful times, leading to a cycle of stress-induced eating and potential negative effects on physical and emotional health. Mindful awareness of stress triggers and adopting healthier coping strategies is essential for maintaining balanced eating habits during challenging times.

Mindful eating techniques to prevent overeating:

1. Slow down: Eat slowly and savour each bite. Put down your utensils between bites and chew thoroughly. This allows your body to

recognise feelings of fullness and prevents overeating.

2. Pay attention: Focus on the flavour's, textures, and aromas of your food. Be present in the moment and avoid distractions like TV or smartphones while eating.

3. Understand your body language: Tune in to your body's hunger and fullness cues. Eat when you're genuinely hungry and stop when you feel satisfied, not overly full.

4. Portion control: Use smaller plates and serving utensils to help control portion sizes. Avoid mindless eating from large containers or bags.

5. Stay hydrated: Sometimes, thirst can be mistaken for hunger. Drink water throughout the day to ensure you are not confusing dehydration with hunger.

6. Avoid emotional eating: Be mindful of emotional triggers that may lead to overeating. Find alternative ways to cope with stress or emotions, such as meditation, going for a walk, or engaging in a hobby.

7. Plan meals and snacks: Prepare balanced

meals and have healthy snacks on hand to avoid reaching for unhealthy options when hunger strikes.

8. Practice mindful food choices: Before eating, ask yourself if you're truly hungry or just eating out of habit or boredom. Choose nutritious foods that nourish your body and mind.

9. Be forgiving: If you do overeat occasionally, don't be too hard on yourself. Practice self-compassion and use the experience as an opportunity to learn and improve mindful eating habits.

By incorporating these mindful eating techniques into your daily routine, you can prevent overeating, develop a healthier relationship with food, and better listen to your body's signals for hunger and fullness.

How to manage stress and emotional eating as a busy professional

As a busy professional, managing stress and emotional eating is essential.

Identify triggers, prioritise self-care, and practice stress management techniques like meditation or yoga. Plan balanced meals and have healthy snacks available to avoid unhealthy choices.

Stay hydrated, practice mindful eating, and seek support if needed.

Remember to be patient with yourself and focus on progress, not perfection. By taking these steps, you can cultivate a healthier relationship with food and effectively manage stress.

Chapter 5

Making Fitness Part of Your Daily Routine

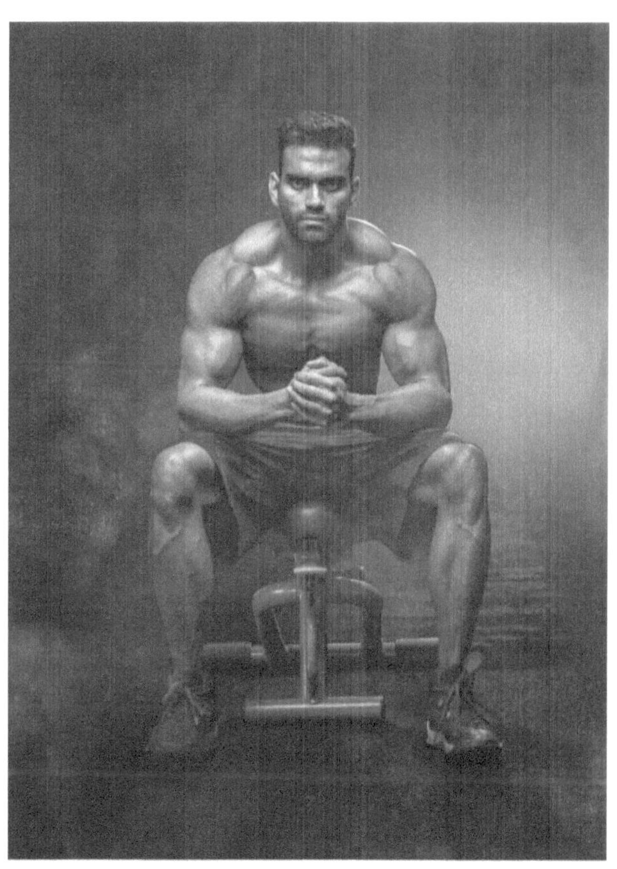

Strategies for integrating physical activity into your workday:

1. Take active breaks: Set reminders to stand up, stretch, or take short walks every hour. These active breaks can help prevent sedentary behaviour and boost energy levels.

2. Walk or bike to work: If feasible, consider walking, biking, or using public transportation part of the way to work. This adds physical activity to your day and reduces stress from commuting.

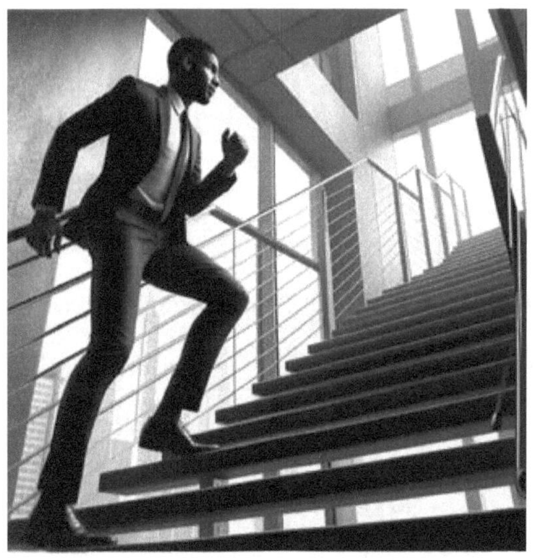

3. Use stairs instead of elevators: Opt for stairs whenever possible. Climbing stairs is an

excellent way to fit in some cardiovascular exercise during your workday.

4. Desk exercises: Incorporate desk exercises like leg lifts, shoulder rolls, or seated twists to keep your muscles active and reduce tension.

5. Stand while working: If possible, use a standing desk or create a makeshift standing workstation by elevating your computer and keyboard. Standing engages core muscles and burns more calories than sitting.

6. Schedule active meetings: Instead of sitting in a conference room, suggest walking meetings or discussions outside. It encourages creativity and adds physical activity to your day.

7. Lunchtime workouts: Utilize your lunch break for a quick workout. Go for a walk, run, or try a short bodyweight exercise routine nearby.

8. Use fitness apps: Download fitness apps that provide short exercise routines or reminders to move throughout the day.

9. Stretch at your desk: Incorporate simple

stretching exercises to relieve tension and stiffness during long work hours.

10. Park farther away: If you drive to work, park farther from the entrance to add extra steps to your day.

11. Take the long route: Choose longer routes when walking to the restroom, breakroom, or other areas of your workplace.

12. Form a fitness group: Encourage colleagues to join a fitness group or start one yourself. Working out together can be motivating and fun.

By integrating these strategies into your workday, you can improve your physical fitness, boost mood, and reduce stress, ultimately leading to a healthier and more productive work-life balance.

Turning household chores into exercise opportunities

As a busy professional, finding time for formal exercise may be challenging. However, you can turn household chores into exercise opportunities to stay active and healthy. Here are some practical ways to do it:

1. Speed cleaning: Amp up the intensity of your cleaning by doing it more quickly. This will increase your heart rate and turn cleaning into a cardio workout.

2. Squat and reach: Incorporate squats as you reach for items while organising shelves or picking up things from the floor. This engages your leg and core muscles.

3. Dance breaks: Take short dance breaks while doing household tasks. Play your favourite tunes and dance around while cooking or doing the dishes to add some fun and movement.

4. Active laundry day: Instead of carrying a full laundry basket, make multiple trips up and down the stairs or around the house. This increases your step count and burns extra calories.

5. Vacuum lunges: While vacuuming, add lunges as you move from one area to another. It's an excellent way to work your legs and add some strength training to your cleaning routine.

6. Wall push-ups: When waiting for something to finish in the kitchen, do wall push-ups

against the counter. It's a quick way to engage your upper body.

7. Calf raises at the sink: While brushing your teeth or washing dishes, do calf raises by lifting your heels off the ground. This helps strengthen your calf muscles.

8. Outdoor chores: Embrace outdoor chores like gardening, mowing the lawn, or raking leaves. These activities provide a full-body workout and fresh air.

9. Multitasking lunges: While talking on the phone or waiting for something to cook, do stationary lunges to target your leg muscles.

10. Core engaging: Engage your core muscles as you move around the house, whether it is walking from room to room or going up and down stairs.

Remember, even small bursts of physical activity add up throughout the day. By incorporating these exercise opportunities into your household chores, you can stay active and maintain your well-being as a busy professional. Be creative and make the most out of your daily routines!

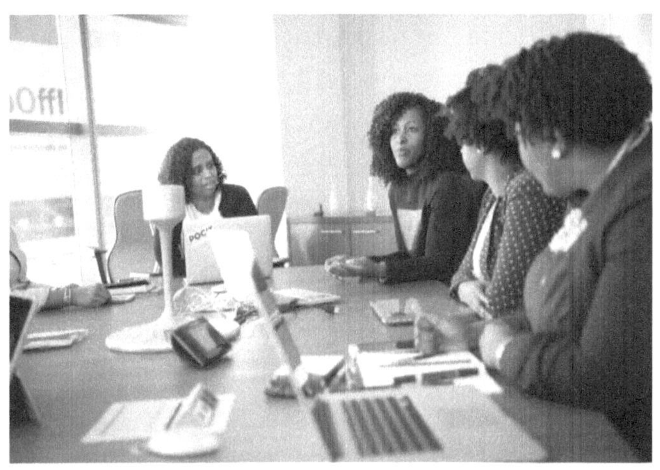

Conclusion

Encouragement to take small steps towards a healthier lifestyle:

Remember, a healthier lifestyle is not about making drastic changes overnight. It is all about taking small, sustainable steps that lead to significant improvements over time.

Below are some encouraging reminders to help you embark on your journey towards a healthier life:

1. Every step counts: Whether it's opting for a piece of fruit instead of a sugary snack or taking a short walk during your lunch break, each small choice contributes to your overall well-being.

2. Celebrate progress: Acknowledge and celebrate every small achievement along the way. Each step you take towards a healthier lifestyle is an accomplishment worth recognising.

3. Embrace consistency: Consistency is key. Small, consistent actions compound over time to create lasting positive changes.

4. Be kind to yourself: Embrace self-compassion and patience. It's okay to stumble; what matters is getting back up and continuing on your journey.

5. Focus on what you can control: Rather than getting overwhelmed by everything you want to change, focus on the things you can control right now. Take it one step at a time.

6. Find joy in the process: Discover activities and healthy choices that bring you joy. When you enjoy what you're doing, it becomes easier to maintain a healthier lifestyle.

7. Set realistic goals: Start with achievable goals that fit into your current lifestyle. As you achieve them, you can gradually set new ones to keep progressing.

8. Build a support system: Surround yourself with supportive friends, family, or online communities that encourage your healthier choices and offer motivation.

9. Learn from setbacks: See setbacks as opportunities for growth. Reflect on what you can learn from them and use that knowledge to move forward.

10. Prioritise sleep: Rest is vital for overall health. Aim for consistent and sufficient sleep to recharge your body and mind.

11. Remember your "Why": Stay connected to your reasons for pursuing a healthier lifestyle. Remind yourself of the benefits you will experience along the way.

12. Enjoy the journey: Embrace the process of becoming healthier, as it's not just about the destination but also about the experiences and discoveries you make along the way. Every small step you take towards a healthier lifestyle matters. Start with one change today, and let it lead you to a more vibrant and fulfilling life.

Final thoughts and motivation for professionals on the move to prioritise fitness and nutrition:

To all busy professionals, remember that your health is your greatest asset. Prioritising fitness and nutrition doesn't require drastic changes; it's about making small, sustainable choices every day. By investing in your well-being, you will have more energy, improved focus, and increased productivity to conquer your professional challenges.

Taking time for regular physical activity and nourishing your body with wholesome foods is an investment in a healthier and happier future. These habits not only benefit your work life but also enhance your personal life, enabling you to be your best self for yourself and your loved ones.

Remember, you deserve to thrive both professionally and personally. Make self-care and well-being a priority, and watch as you unlock your full potential and achieve success in all aspects of your life. Your health is worth it, and you are worth it.

Start today, take one small step at a time, and let your commitment to fitness and nutrition propel you towards a fulfilling and prosperous future.

Cheers!